The XXL Low Carb Cookbook for UK

Quick and Delicious Recipes for Every Day incl. 14 Days LC Challenge for Sustainable Weight Loss

Food Club UK

ISBN- 9798720891275

TABLE OF CONTENTS

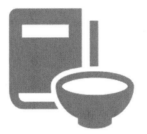

INTRODUCTION

Everyone wants to look and feel their best. It's human nature and by finding a lifestyle that suits you, you can not only achieve those two aims but also strive towards ultimate health at the same time.

You'll no doubt know that fad diets are rife. Perhaps you've followed a few yourself or maybe you've watched from afar and wondered how people actually manage to stick to them. The truth is that they generally don't stick to them at all.

Fad diets are unsustainable, unhealthy, and leave you feeling miserable. They don't give your body the nutrition it really needs and, in the end, you find it almost impossible to stick to the rigid calorie counting required. From weighing your ingredients into small amounts or only eating specific food groups, all of this is unhealthy.

For that reason, it's important to find a weight loss diet which you can stick to. The best advice? Avoid the word 'diet' altogether and instead stick to the phrase 'lifestyle change'.

If you want to lose weight and keep it off, you need to dedicate yourself to changing your lifestyle for the rest of your days. You need to enjoy your favourite unhealthy foods in moderation only and stick to healthy options for the majority of the time. You also need to stop smoking, drink more water, and of course, exercise regularly.

It sounds difficult but it's actually not. The more you focus on a healthy lifestyle, the more addictive it becomes, simply because it feels so good.

This book is going to talk about a specific type of lifestyle change, namely one which requires you to reduce the amount of carbohydrates you eat. It's not a fad diet and it's not unhealthy, although you do need to proceed with caution if you have any specific health concerns – we'll get onto that later!

For now, let's learn more about what a low carb diet actually is.

What is a Low Carb Diet?

There's that word again – 'diet'! What you'll notice from following this healthy eating routine is that you don't struggle with the same downside as you would with a fad diet. Cutting down on the number of carbs you eat isn't in the fad category.

Put simply, this type of eating routine requires you to eat less carbohydrates. To make up for that, you eat a little more fat (natural fats and not artificial ones), and plenty of protein. You might have heard of the Ketogenic Diet, or the Keto Diet, and that's the same thing.

By lowering your carbs, eating a little more natural fat to keep you fuller for longer, getting enough protein, and reducing your sugar intake, you'll lose weight, keep it off, notice you have more energy, and you'll feel great too.

It's actually very easy once you get into it!

There are a few rules to this type of lifestyle:

- Reduce your carb intake by being mindful of how many carbs you're consuming
- Eat more natural fats
- Avoid low fat products as these will just leave you feeling hungry
- Stop eating when you're full
- Drink enough water every day

DON'T COUNT CALORIES OR WEIGH OUT YOUR FOOD INGREDIENTS

- Eat more protein every day
- Stick to foods like meat, eggs, natural fats, fish, and vegetables
- Avoid foods such as pasta, rice, potatoes, bread, beans, and anything sugary
- Enjoy cheat foods only in moderation
- Measure net carbs only, and you should aim to consume no more than 50-100g net carbs per day

It really is as easy as it sounds.

A Word About Ketosis

To understand how minimising your carbohydrate intake works and how it helps you to lose weight and keep it off, you also need to know about a metabolic state called ketosis.

Carbohydrates are used by your body for energy. They're broken down and used to help your internal organs function, give you plenty of natural energy, and to ensure that your body runs in a healthy and efficient way. Now, you might wonder what happens if you reduce carb intake, because surely that means you lack the energy you need.

Not so. Instead, your body starts to burn existing fat stores for energy, and the natural fats that you're eating in your daily routine. This means that you lose existing weight quite quickly and by sticking to the routine, you keep it off. You then burn the fat in your diet to give you the energy you need and to help your body function healthily and smoothly.

In order for this to happen, your body goes into a state called ketosis. At first glance, ketosis sounds unhealthy but stick with the explanation because as long as you follow the rules of a low carb lifestyle, it's not healthy for most people.

Ketosis occurs when your body falsely believes that it's going to starve. When you cut the amount of carbohydrates you're eating, your body panics because it's not sure what it's going to burn for energy. The red alarm is sounded and your brain kicks into survival mode. It turns the fat burning switch on, meaning that your body goes into ketosis.

Ketones are proteins which are produced by the body when it is in the ketosis state. These ketones are burnt for fuel and energy, and they require a higher fat content to be produced. As long as you keep your carbohydrate level low enough for ketosis, you'll stay in this state and the fat burning switch stays on.

However, the problems occur when you dip in and out of it. That means you increase your carb intake one day and then drop it the next. That's when ketosis isn't the safest, because your body is totally confused. So, if you're going to dedicate yourself to following a low carb diet, you need to stick to it over the long-term and not move in and out however the mood takes you.

It's important to note that when you first enter ketosis, you might feel a little under the weather. Unless the symptoms are particularly troublesome to you, you should stick with it. They should ease after two weeks at the most and then you will start to notice the advantages of a low carb diet, which we'll talk about in more detail shortly.

A few signs your body has entered ketosis are:

- Bad breath

- Feeling low in energy for a while, before this picks up and actually makes you feel like you have more energy

- Headaches

- Needing to urinate more often

- Muscle spasms and cramps

- Loss of weight

- Feeling thirsty

You can overcome some of these symptoms by drinking more water and adding salt to your food. However, if you really can't handle the side effects of the first week or two, you should stop the diet and speak to your doctor.

Not all low carb lifestyles push you into ketosis, however in order for it to be most effective, ketosis really needs to be part of the deal.

The Advantages & Disadvantages of a Low Carb Diet

So, what's in it for you? What do you get from not eating your favourite type of bread?

Let's check out the pros and cons of a low carb lifestyle.

Advantages of Low Carb Lifestyles

- Weight loss

- May help to lower cholesterol levels

- Less cravings

- Helps to regulate blood sugar spikes

- May contribute towards better heart health

- More energy

- Better focus and concentration

- Increased quality of sleep

Disadvantages of Low Carb Lifestyles

- Not suitable for absolutely everyone

- Possible vitamin deficiencies if you don't vary your foods and follow the guidance

- Symptoms of ketosis at the start can be troublesome

- Challenging at the start

- Gut health may suffer if you're prone to stomach problems. In that case, taking a probiotic supplement may help but again, gain advice from your doctor first

Every lifestyle change or diet has its pros and cons and the low carb option is no different. However, as you can see, the pros are very advantageous and the cons are either not going to affect you or they can be reduced in severity.

Who Shouldn't Follow a Low Carb Diet?

Whilst a low carb diet is relatively safe for anyone, there are some people who need to be a little more cautious and speak to their doctor before they start.

If you're taking medication for diabetes, if you're breastfeeding or pregnant, and if you're taking any other medications, then you should speak to your doctor and heed their advice. It may be that in some cases, e.g. if you're diabetic, you need to tweak the diet a little to ensure safety and diabetes control. For that reason, stick to your doctor's advice.

For pregnant and breastfeeding women, the advice is a little unclear. The best route is to perhaps wait until the baby is born and you've finished breastfeeding, before cutting down your carbs. That way, you've covered all safety bases.

In addition, anyone who has any kidney or liver issues should also discuss the possibility of low carb diets with their doctor. In some cases, low carb options may not be for you.

However, for most people, this is a positive choice to make and one which will bring you many advantages. If you're not sure, simply have a chat with your doctor and get the green light before you begin.

Are You Ready?

The low carb lifestyle isn't a difficult one once you get into the swing of it. It takes some getting used to, that's for sure, but it's a lifestyle change that will certainly help you to lose weight and keep it off.

Many fad diets help you to lose weight, and in some cases, it can be quite a lot at the start, but as soon as you start eating normally again, the weight comes straight back on. When you dedicate yourself to a low carb diet, you'll find that you eat normally by simply avoiding foods which are high in carbs and you won't feel hungry because of the high natural fat content and protein.

The rest of the book will help you to understand how a low carb diet works and we're going to give you plenty of inspiration in terms of what to cook and how to do it. In addition, you'll find a 14 day meal plan at the end of the book, giving you support over the first two weeks of your new lifestyle change.

All that's left to do is to get started!

LOW CARBOHYDRATE RECIPES

The great news is that it's far easier than you might think to recreate fantastic and delicious recipes that are low in carbohydrate content. In this section, you'll find countless recipes to try for yourself, with ingredients that can easily be found in supermarkets. You might not have heard of erythritol or psyllium husk before, but believe us, they're in the supermarket and they're more popular than you might think!

You'll find a range of breakfast dishes, lunches, and dinners, as well as a bonus section of desserts. We've mixed meat and vegetarian options and you'll soon see how flexible and interchangeable many of the recipes are.

To make life a little easier, why not plan your meals the day before or follow the meal plan a little later in the book? That way, you can purchase all the ingredients you need, take advantage of supermarket offers, save money, and also save time. You can also make many of these recipes ahead and refrigerate or freeze them to enjoy later.

The low carb lifestyle is flexible, easy to follow, and it fits in perfectly with a busy lifestyle.

Breakfasts

Low carb breakfasts revolve heavily around eggs, because they're so filling and easy to cook. However, you'll also find several other recipes in this section which are egg-free and super-easy to make.

Easy Bacon & Eggs

Serves 4
Fat – 32g, Net carbs – 1g, Protein – 20g, Calories – 377

INGREDIENTS

- ♦ 8 medium eggs
- ♦ 260g bacon
- ♦ A handful of cherry tomatoes

METHOD

1. Take a medium frying pan and cook your bacon to your preferred level
2. Place the bacon to one side but keep the fat in the pan
3. Crack your eggs into the frying pan with the bacon fat and cook them to your desired level
4. Halve your cherry tomatoes and fry them for a few minutes to serve alongside

Buttery Scrambled Eggs

Serves 1
Fat – 61g, Net carbs – 3g, Protein – 25g, Calories – 657

INGREDIENTS

- ◆ 2 medium eggs
- ◆ 55g grated cheese, cheddar works best
- ◆ 2 tbsp butter
- ◆ 2 tbsp basil, fresh
- ◆ 2 tbsp double cream
- ◆ Salt and pepper for seasoning

METHOD

1. Take a medium frying pan and add the butter over a medium heat, until melted
2. In a small mixing bowl, add the eggs, cheese, and cream and combine with a little seasoning
3. Pour the mixture into the pan and swirl it around to coat the pan
4. Use a plastic spatula to move the eggs away from the edges of the pan and keep them unstuck
5. Cook until the eggs are how you like them
6. Serve with a little basil over the top

Classic Huevos Rancheros

Serves 4
Fat – 47g, Net carbs – 12g, Protein – 17g, Calories – 547

INGREDIENTS

- 120ml extra virgin olive oil
- 2 minced cloves of garlic
- 2 minced jalapeno peppers
- 1 minced onion
- 8 medium eggs
- 1 can of crushed tomatoes
- Salt and pepper for seasoning

METHOD

1. Take a medium saucepan and add a third of the oil
2. Add the peppers and cook over a medium heat until they soften
3. Add the garlic and the onion and combine
4. Cook for a few minutes, until the onions are soft
5. Add the tomatoes and turn the heat down to a simmer
6. Cover the pan until a thicker sauce has formed
7. Add a little salt and pepper, combine, and remove the pan from the heat
8. Take a frying pan and add the rest of the oil
9. Fry your eggs to your liking and season
10. Place your eggs on a plate and add the tomato sauce on the side

Fruity Strawberry Breakfast Smoothie

Serves 2
Fat – 42g, Net carbs – 10g, Protein – 4g, Calories – 416

INGREDIENTS

- 140g sliced strawberries, fresh work best
- Half a teaspoon of vanilla extract
- 425ml coconut milk
- 1 tbsp fresh lime juice

METHOD

1. Take a blender and add all ingredients to the main section
2. Give everything a quick stir and then blend to your desired thickness
3. Give it a taste and if you like, you can add a little more lime juice

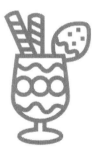

Cheesy Scrambled Eggs With Spinach

Serves 2
Fat – 30g, Net carbs – 4g, Protein – 16g, Calories – 348

INGREDIENTS

- 2 tbsp double cream
- 4 medium eggs
- 1 minced garlic clove
- 45g crumbled feta cheese
- 2 tbsp butter
- 110g baby spinach, fresh
- Salt and pepper for seasoning

METHOD

1. Take a medium mixing bowl and add the cream and eggs, combining well
2. Take a large frying pan and add the butter over a medium heat
3. Add the spinach and the garlic and cook for a few minutes
4. Season with salt and pepper and combine well
5. Add the eggs into the frying pan and allow to cook around the edges
6. Use a spatula to move the eggs from the edges a little and cook until the eggs are how you like them
7. Add the cheese to the top of the eggs and remove from the heat

Spinach Breakfast Frittata

Serves 4

Fat – 60g, Net carbs – 4g, Protein – 27g, Calories – 669

INGREDIENTS

- 2 tbsp butter
- 8 medium eggs
- 240ml double cream
- 140g bacon, diced
- 230g spinach, fresh works best
- 140g grated cheddar cheese
- Salt and pepper for seasoning

METHOD

1. Take a medium baking dish and grease the inside
2. Preheat the oven to 175°C
3. Take a medium frying pan and cook the bacon with the butter until it is how you like it
4. Add the spinach into the pan and combine until it is wilted
5. Take the pan and set it to one side
6. Take a small mixing bowl and combine the cream and eggs
7. Pour into the baking dish
8. Add the bacon and spinach mixture to the baking dish and combine
9. Place into the oven for around 25 minutes, until golden

Blueberry Pancakes

Serves 4
Fat – 43g, Net carbs – 6g, Protein – 15g, Calories – 468

INGREDIENTS

- 85g butter, melted
- 6 medium eggs
- 85g blueberries, fresh work best
- 110g cream cheese
- 160ml oat fibre
- 2 tsp baking powder
- 160ml almond flour
- The zest of half a lemon

METHOD

1. Take a medium mixing bowl and add the cream cheese, butter, and eggs. Combine together well
2. Add all the other ingredients one by one and combine, except for the fresh blueberries
3. Set the batter to one side for five minutes
4. Take a medium frying pan (non-stick) and add a little batter at a time, cooking for a few minutes on one side
5. Flip the pancakes over and cook for another few minutes

6. Before the pancake is completely firm, add a few blueberries but do not press down

7. Cook for another minute, until golden brown

8. Serve whilst still warm

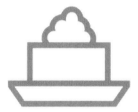

Cheesy Omelette

Serves 2
Fat – 80g, Net carbs – 4g, Protein – 40g, Calories – 895

INGREDIENTS

- ◆ 6 medium eggs
- ◆ 200g grated cheese
- ◆ 85g butter
- ◆ Salt and pepper for seasoning

METHOD

1. Take a medium mixing bowl and add the eggs, whisk until you see a froth start to form
2. Add half of the cheese and season with salt and pepper, combining well
3. Add the butter to a frying pan and melt
4. Add the eggs and cook for a few minutes
5. Turn down the heat and add the rest of the cheese when the egg is nearly cooked
6. Fold the omelette over and serve

Cauliflower Breakfast Pancakes

Serves 4
Fat – 26g, Net carbs – 5g, Protein – 7g, Calories – 282

INGREDIENTS

- 3 medium eggs
- Half a grated onion
- 450g cauliflower
- 110g butter
- Salt and pepper for seasoning

METHOD

1. Place the cauliflower into a food processor and pulse until it resembles a fine consistency. Alternatively, you can use a grater
2. Take a large mixing bowl and add the cauliflower, along with the rest of the ingredients, except for the butter. Combine well
3. Take a large frying pan and add the butter until melted
4. Take a handful of the cauliflower mixture and form it into a ball, flattening it down into a patty, placing it into the frying pan and cooking for 5 minutes on each side
5. Repeat with the rest of the mixture
6. Cook until golden brown and serve warm

Egg Muffins

Serves 6
Fat – 27g, Net carbs – 2g, Protein – 21g, Calories – 335

INGREDIENTS

- ◆ 12 medium eggs
- ◆ 2 chopped scallions
- ◆ 2 tsp pesto
- ◆ 170g grated cheddar cheese
- ◆ 140g bacon, cooked and chopped
- ◆ Salt and pepper for seasoning

METHOD

1. Take a muffin tin and grease the insides with butter
2. Preheat the oven to 175°C
3. Add a little bacon to the bottom of each muffin tin
4. Add a few chopped scallions to the bottom of each muffin tin
5. Take a mixing bowl and add the eggs and pesto, combining well. Season and combine once more
6. Add a little of the egg mixture to each of the muffin tins
7. Add a little cheese to the top of each muffin tin
8. Bake in the oven for 20 minutes, but check after 15 minutes to ensure the muffins aren't burning

Lunches

Traditional Caesar Salad

Make these delicious recipes fresh for your lunchtime meal, or make them ahead of time and keep them in the refrigerator until your break at work. Many can be eaten cold, and several you can warm up. However, be sure to warm up meat until very hot in the middle and be cautious with fish.

Serves 2

Fat – 88g, Net carbs – 4g, Protein – 55g, Calories – 1044

INGREDIENTS

- ♦ 20g grated Parmesan
- ♦ 1 tbsp Dijon mustard
- ♦ 1 finely chopped garlic clove
- ♦ 120ml mayonnaise
- ♦ 2 tbsp chopped anchovies
- ♦ Zest and juice of half a lemon
- ♦ Salt and pepper for seasoning
- ♦ 350g chicken breasts
- ♦ 1 tbsp olive oil
- ♦ 200g chopped lettuce
- ♦ 40g shredded Parmesan
- ♦ 85g cooked bacon, chopped

1. Place the mayonnaise, mustard, grated Parmesan, anchovies and garlic into a bowl and either whisk or use a blender to create a dressing. Place to one side
2. Preheat your oven to 175°C
3. Take a large baking dish and grease the inside
4. Add the chicken breasts to the baking dish and season
5. Drizzle a little olive oil over the top of the chicken and bake until cooked, around 20 minutes
6. Once cooled, slice the chicken
7. Take your plates and add the lettuce first, before adding slices of the chicken
8. Add the chopped bacon on top
9. Drizzle the dressing over the top of the plate and add a little of the remaining parmesan to serve

Healthy Avocado & Salmon

Serves 2

Fat – 45g, Net carbs – 4g, Protein – 25g, Calories – 548

INGREDIENTS

- 2 avocados
- 2 tbsp mayonnaise
- 230g smoked salmon
- Salt and pepper for seasoning

METHOD

1. Cut each avocado in half and remove the pit. Use a spoon to scoop out the avocado flesh and put onto your plate
2. Arrange the smoked salmon next to the avocado
3. Add mayonnaise either on top, or on the side
4. Season and enjoy!

Tuna & Boiled Eggs

Serves 2
Fat – 76g, Net carbs – 3g, Protein – 52g, Calories – 930

INGREDIENTS

- 55g spinach, cooked
- 1 avocado
- 4 medium eggs
- 1 can of tuna in oil
- 120ml mayonnaise
- Salt and pepper for seasoning

METHOD

1. Boil your eggs to your liking and place them to one side to cool
2. Cut your avocados into halves and remove the pit. Use a spoon to scoop out the flesh and place it onto your plate
3. Add the cooked spinach next to the avocado
4. Remove the shells from the eggs and cut into halves
5. Place the eggs onto the plate and season

Halloumi With Mushrooms

Serves 2
Fat – 72g, Net carbs – 803g, Protein – 34g, Calories – 803

INGREDIENTS

♦ 280g halloumi cheese

♦ 280g mushrooms

♦ A handful of olives

♦ 85g butter

♦ Salt and pepper for seasoning

♦ Butter for frying

METHOD

1. Slice the mushrooms to your desired size
2. Take a large frying pan and add the butter, melting over a medium heat
3. Add the mushrooms to the pan and fry for around 5 minutes
4. Season and combine
5. Add the halloumi to the pan and cook for a few minutes on each side, stirring the mushrooms at the same time
6. Turn the heat down a little and add the olives for the last minute or so

Avocado & Tuna Salad

Serves 4
Fat – 45g, Net carbs – 7g, Protein – 44g, Calories – 639

INGREDIENTS

- ◆ 3 avocados, pitted and sliced into pieces
- ◆ 1 can of tuna in oil
- ◆ 80ml olive oil
- ◆ 2 tbsp fresh lime juice
- ◆ 1 cucumber, cut into quarters
- ◆ 1 red onion, cut into slices
- ◆ 2 red bell peppers, cut into slices
- ◆ Salt and pepper for seasoning

METHOD

1. Drain the tuna and use a fork to divide the meat into flaky pieces
2. Add the avocado, cucumber, onion, and peppers to the serving bowl and mix together
3. Add the tuna and mix with the other ingredients
4. Take a small mixing bowl and combine the lemon juice with the olive oil and create a dressing
5. Drizzle the dressing over the salad and season to your liking

Tasty Baked Eggs

Serves 1
Fat – 37g, Net carbs – 1g, Protein – 41g, Calories – 509

INGREDIENTS

- ◆ 2 medium eggs
- ◆ 55g grated cheese
- ◆ 85g ground beef

METHOD

1. Take a small baking dish and lightly grease the inside
2. Preheat your oven to 200°C
3. Add the ground beef to the baking dish and flatten it to create a layer
4. Add two holes in the beef, where you will add the eggs
5. Crack one egg into each hole
6. Add the cheese over the whole dish equally
7. Season to your liking
8. Place the dish into the oven and bake for 15 minutes
9. Allow to cool slightly before serving

Healthy Green Beans With Salmon

Serves 2
Fat – 58g, Net carbs – 6g, Protein – 38g, Calories – 705

INGREDIENTS

- 85g butter
- 350g salmon fillets, boneless
- 250g green beans, fresh
- The juice of half a lemon
- Salt and pepper for seasoning

METHOD

1. Take the green beans and trim them down to your liking
2. Take a large frying pan and melt the butter over a medium heat
3. Add the salmon to the pan and the green beans alongside
4. Cook the salmon for around 4 minutes on each side
5. Turn the beans at the halfway point
6. Season with salt and pepper to your liking
7. Just before the fish has finished cooking, add the lemon juice over the whole pan

Lunchtime Chicken Soup

Serves 8
Fat – 40g, Net carbs – 4g, Protein – 33g, Calories – 508

INGREDIENTS

- 1 ½ rotisserie chicken
- 110g butter
- 5 sliced carrots
- 2 minced onions
- 170g sliced onions
- 2 chopped celery stalks
- 140g sliced green cabbage
- 2 garlic cloves, minced
- 2 litres of chicken broth
- 2 tsp parsley, dried
- Salt and pepper for seasoning

METHOD

1. Take a large saucepan and add the butter, melting it over a medium heat
2. Add the mushrooms, celery, garlic, and onions and combine well, cooking for 4 minutes
3. Add the carrots, parsley, broth and seasoning and combine
4. Simmer the mixture until the vegetables are soft

5. Meanwhile, shred the rotisserie chicken with two forks
6. Add the cabbage and combine
7. Add the chicken and combine once more
8. Simmer the mixture for 12 minutes, until everything is tender

Halloumi Bacon Wraps

Serves 2

Fat – 59g, Net carbs – 3g, Protein – 35g, Calories – 684

INGREDIENTS

- ◆ 170g sliced bacon, cut into 10 pieces
- ◆ 230g halloumi cheese

METHOD

1. Take the halloumi and cut it into 10 pieces, making sure they're all as even as possible
2. Preheat your oven to 225°C
3. Take a baking sheet and line it with parchment paper
4. Pick up a piece of cheese and wrap one piece of bacon around it, folding the edge underneath to stop it from coming undone in the oven
5. Repeat with the rest of the cheese and bacon
6. Place the bacon wrapped cheese onto the baking tray and bake in the oven for 15 minutes, turning halfway

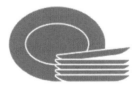

Crispy Bacon With Fried Cabbage

Serves 2
Fat – 76g, Net carbs – 8g, Protein – 23g, Calories – 816

INGREDIENTS

- 55g butter
- 450g green cabbage
- 280g bacon
- Salt and pepper for seasoning

METHOD

1. Cut the cabbage into small pieces and repeat the process with the bacon
2. Take a large frying pan and melt the butter over a medium heat
3. Cook the bacon until it is as crispy as you like it
4. Add the cabbage to the pan just before the bacon is done and cook until crispy
5. Season and serve

Dinners

A hearty and filling dinner will keep those late night cravings away, and will help you to avoid unhealthy snacking later in the evening. Below you'll find a range of meals with meats, fish, and vegetarian choices. Most are quite quick to make too, so as long as you have the ingredients to hand, you can rustle up a delicious meal when you return home from work.

Fragrant Garlic Chicken

Serves 4

Fat – 39g, Net carbs – 3g, Protein – 42g, Calories – 540

INGREDIENTS

- 900g chicken drumsticks
- Juice of 1 lemon
- 55g butter
- 30g chopped fresh parsley
- 2 tbsp olive oil
- 7 sliced cloves of garlic
- Salt and pepper for seasoning

METHOD

1. Take a large baking tray and grease with butter
2. Preheat the oven to 225 °C
3. Arrange the chicken drumsticks onto the tray and add salt and pepper to season
4. In a small mixing bowl, combine the oil and lemon juice
5. Drizzle the oil mixture over the chicken liberally
6. Sprinkle the parsley and the garlic over the chicken
7. Cook in the oven for around 40 minutes, ensuring the chicken is cooked properly

Low Carb Chicken Korma

Serves 4
Fat – 31g, Net carbs – 3g, Protein – 34g, Calories – 440

INGREDIENTS

- 650g chicken drumsticks
- 110g Greek yogurt
- 60ml ghee
- Half an onion, cut into slices
- 1 bay leaf
- 1 star anise
- 3 cloves
- 1 stick of cinnamon
- 8 black peppercorns
- 3 cardamom pods
- 1 tsp red chilli powder
- Half a tsp ginger paste
- Half a tsp turmeric
- 1 tsp coriander seeds, ground
- 1 tsp cumin, ground
- Half a tsp garam masala
- Salt and pepper for seasoning

METHOD

1. Take a large saucepan and add the ghee until melted
2. Add the onions and fry over a medium heat until golden
3. Transfer the onions onto a plate and set aside, keeping the ghee in the pan
4. Add the yogurt into a blender and add the onions, pulse until creamy
5. Turn the heat back on and reheat the ghee
6. Add the bay leaf, cinnamon, cloves, cardamom, star anise, and peppercorns, cooking for 30 seconds
7. Add the chicken and season
8. Add the garlic paste and give everything a good stir, cooking for 2 minutes
9. Add the coriander powder, garam masala, turmeric, red chilli powder and the cumin, stirring everything well and cooking for a further 2 minutes
10. Pour the yogurt paste over the top of the thicken and give everything a good stir. If it's too thick, add a little water to loosen it
11. Cover the pan and cook for 15 minutes, ensuring the chicken is cooked through

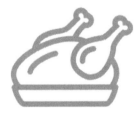

Lasagne With Courgette

Serves 6
Fat – 53g, Net carbs – 7g, Protein – 34g, Calories – 644

INGREDIENTS

- 650g ground beef
- 2 tbsp olive oil
- 400g sliced courgette
- 1 chopped onion
- 2 chopped garlic cloves
- 4 tbsp tomato paste
- 1 tbsp basil, dried
- 1 tbsp oregano, dried
- Quarter a tsp black pepper
- 3 tbsp cold water
- 350ml double cream
- 1 minced garlic clove
- 230g grated cheese
- Salt and pepper for seasoning

METHOD

1. Take a large baking dish and preheat your oven to 200°C
2. Take the courgette and season with salt, placing to one side for a short while
3. Take a large pan and add the oil, heating over a medium heat
4. Add the garlic and onion and cook until soft

5. Add the meat, oregano, basil, and season

6. Combine everything together and cook until the meat is browned

7. Add the tomato paste and combine once more

8. Turn the temperature down just a little, stir well, and allow to simmer for 10 minutes

9. Take a medium saucepan and add the cream, garlic, and half of the grated cheese, stirring well

10. Allow to simmer and once it starts to bubble more, turn the heat down and simmer for another 5 minutes, stirring as you go

11. Season the sauce and stir until thick

12. Take the baking dish and add a third of the meat over the bottom

13. Add a little of the cheese sauce as the next layer

14. Add the courgette slices side by side to cover the top layer

15. Repeat the meat, cheese, and courgette routine until you reach the top of the baking dish

16. Bake for 20 minutes and allow to sit for around 15 minutes before you serve

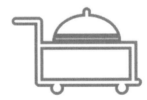

Goat's Cheese & Spinach Dinner Pie

Serves 6
Fat – 57g, Net carbs – 4g, Protein – 23g, Calories – 636

INGREDIENTS

- ♦ 45g butter
- ♦ 1 medium egg (for the crust)
- ♦ 140g almond flour
- ♦ 1 tbsp psyllium husk powder, ground
- ♦ 3 tbsp sesame seeds
- ♦ 5 medium eggs (for the batter)
- ♦ 240ml double cream
- ♦ 2 tbsp coconut oil
- ♦ 1 chopped garlic clove
- ♦ 1 tsp nutmeg, ground
- ♦ 200g chopped fresh spinach
- ♦ 110g grated cheese (cheddar works well)
- ♦ 170g sliced goat's cheese
- ♦ Salt and pepper for seasoning

METHOD

1. Preheat your oven to 175°C
2. Take a blender and add the sesame seeds and the almond flour, combining well
3. Add the butter, psyllium husk powder, 1 egg and a little salt and combine together until a dough forms

4. Take a large springform pan and press the dough into the bottom and up the sides
5. Prick holes along the base of the pie dough
6. Cook in the oven for 15 minutes, checking after 10 minutes to ensure it isn't burning
7. Take a mixing bowl and combine the remaining eggs and cream
8. Season and combine once more
9. Take a medium frying pan and add the oil to a medium heat
10. Add the garlic and sauté
11. Add the spinach and cook until wilted
12. Add the spinach to the pie shell and evenly distribute
13. Add the cheese to the egg mixture and combine
14. Pour the mixture over the top of the spinach
15. Arrange the sliced goat's cheese over the top
16. Place the pie in the oven and cook for 40 minutes

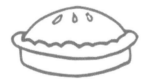

Creamy Cauliflower Cheese

Serves 6

Fat – 46g, Net carbs – 12g, Protein – 17g, Calories – 527

INGREDIENTS

- 200g cream cheese
- 450g broccoli florets, fresh or frozen
- 800g cauliflower florets
- 240ml double cream
- 2 tsp garlic powder
- 55g butter, plus extra for greasing
- 230g grated cheese
- Salt and pepper for seasoning

METHOD

1. Take a large baking dish and grease with a little butter
2. Preheat the oven to 180°C
3. Take a large saucepan and add the broccoli
4. Add enough water to cover the broccoli and allow to boil, before turning the temperature down and cooking until tender
5. Strain the broccoli and add the cream, cream cheese, garlic powder, butter and seasoning to the pan and combine everything well
6. Use an immersion blender to create a puree

7. Add the broccoli and blend once more until you have a smooth mixture

8. Arrange the cauliflower inside the baking dish

9. Pour the sauce over the cauliflower and sprinkle the cheese over the top

10. Cook in the oven for 40 minutes

Low Carb Chowder

Serves 4
Fat – 69g, Net carbs – 6g, Protein – 37g, Calories – 792

INGREDIENTS

- 240ml clam juice
- 450g boneless salmon fillets, cut into pieces of around 1 inch size
- 230g peeled and deveined shrimp
- 2 minced garlic cloves
- 4 tbsp butter
- 110g cream cheese
- 350ml double cream
- 140g sliced celery
- The juice and zest of half a lemon
- 2 tsp thyme, dried
- 55g baby spinach
- Half a tbsp red chilli powder

METHOD

1. Take a large saucepan and add the butter over a medium heat
2. Once the butter has melted, add the celery and garlic and cook for 5 minutes
3. Add the cream cheese, cream, clam juice, zest and lemon juice, combining well
4. Simmer for around 10 minutes, uncovered to ensure the juice doesn't disappear

5. Add the shrimp and the fish and combine
6. Simmer for 3 minutes, checking that the fish is cooked
7. Add the spinach and cook until it has wilted, stirring regularly
8. Season with a little salt and pepper
9. Serve with the red chili and sage on the plate

Creamy Tuna Casserole

Serves 4
Fat – 45g, Net carbs – 5g, Protein – 37g, Calories – 590

INGREDIENTS

- 1 can of drained tuna
- 28g butter
- 375g celery stalks
- 1 onion
- 1 green bell pepper
- 80g grated parmesan cheese
- 180ml mayonnaise
- 1 tsp chili flakes
- Salt and pepper for seasoning

METHOD

1. Take a large baking dish and grease the inside with butter, placing it to one side
2. Preheat the oven to 200°C
3. Chop the bell pepper, celery, and the onion finely
4. Take a large frying pan and add the butter until melted
5. Fry the onion, celery, and pepper until soft, adding a little salt and pepper as seasoning

6. Add the mayonnaise, tuna, parmesan and chili flakes into the baking dish and combine well

7. Add the vegetables and combine once more

8. Place in the oven for 15 minutes

Meatball & Bacon Casserole

Serves 4
Fat – 75g, Net carbs – 6g, Protein – 47g, Calories – 898

INGREDIENTS

- 450g ground beef
- 200g diced bacon
- 2 tins of diced tomatoes
- 1 minced garlic clove
- 2 chopped dill pickles
- 230g grated cheese
- 2 medium eggs
- 2 tbsp tomato ketchup
- 240ml double cream
- Salt and pepper for seasoning

METHOD

1. Take a large casserole dish and preheat the oven to 200 °C
2. Take a large frying pan and add the bacon, cooking until it is as crispy as you like it
3. Move the bacon to one side but keep the fat in the pan
4. Add the beef and turn up the heat
5. Fry until the meat is brown and cooked
6. Add the tomatoes and the pickles and combine
7. Add the garlic, most of the cheese, and season with salt and pepper

8. Transfer the meat mixture to the casserole dish and add the bacon, combining well
9. Take a small mixing bowl and add the cream, tomato ketchup and the eggs, combining well
10. Pour the egg over the meat and sprinkle with the remaining cheese
11. Place in the oven and cook for 25 minutes

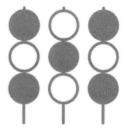

Homemade Low Carb Pizza

Serves 2

Fat – 86g, Net carbs – 6g, Protein – 56g, Calories – 1024

INGREDIENTS

- 170g grated mozzarella cheese
- 4 medium eggs
- 170g provolone cheese, shredded
- 3 tbsp tomato sauce
- 45g pepperoni
- 1 tsp oregano, dried
- Salt and pepper for seasoning

METHOD

1. Take a large baking tray and line it with parchment paper
2. Preheat the oven to 200°C
3. Take a medium mixing bowl and add the eggs and half of the mozzarella cheese
4. Combine well to create a sticky dough
5. Using a plastic spatula, create a round shape on the parchment. You can do one large one, or two smaller ones – it's up to you!
6. Place the baking tray in the oven for 15 minutes, until the crust is a little brown
7. Place to one side for a couple of minutes, but keep the oven on
8. Once cooled slightly, add the tomato sauce on top of the pizza crust and spread to coat

9. Add a little oregano on top and add the rest of the cheeses, distributing evenly

10. Add the pepperoni on top and season to your liking

11. Place back in the oven for another 10 minutes, until the cheese has melted

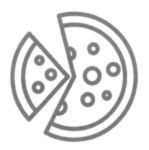

Cauliflower Mash & Steak

Serves 4
Fat – 84g, Net carbs – 10g, Protein – 55g, Calories – 1014

INGREDIENTS

- 800g ribeye steak
- 1 tbsp ghee
- 2 crushed garlic cloves
- 1 tbsp butter (for the steak)
- 55g butter (for the mash)
- 650g cauliflower florets
- 110g chopped bacon
- 110g grated cheddar cheese
- 110g cream cheese
- 120ml sour cream
- 33ml sliced scallions
- Salt and pepper for seasoning

METHOD

1. Take a large baking dish and preheat your oven to 200°C
2. Fill a large saucepan with water and lightly salt it
3. Bring the pan to a boil over a high heat
4. Add the cauliflower and bring to the boil, cooking until the cauliflower is tender
5. Strain the cauliflower and place to one side

6. Use an immersion blender to combine the butter, cream cheese, and cauliflower to create a smooth mixture

7. Season and combine once more

8. Take a large frying pan and cook the bacon for around 10 minutes, until it's crispy

9. Remove the bacon and blot on paper towels

10. Add the mixture to the baking dish and sprinkle with the cheese on top, adding the bacon last

11. Place in the oven for around 15 minutes and then place to one side to cool

12. Take the steak and season on both sides

13. Take a large frying pan and add the ghee, cooking the steak over a high heat

14. Add the butter and garlic after a couple of minutes of cooking, and keep ladling the garlic sauce over the steaks as they cook

15. Cook for 5 minutes on each side, until the steak is cooked to your liking

16. Remove the steaks and place them onto a board, covering with foil for around 10 minutes

17. Plate the cauliflower mash and sprinkle with scallions and sour cream, combining well

18. Cut the steak into slices and serve alongside the mash

BONUS – DESSERTS

Good news! You don't have to miss desserts if you have a sweet tooth! There are many low carb-friendly dishes you can make for dessert and many of them are direct copies of the high carb choices you may have had in the past.

There's no reason why you can't enjoy chocolate cake, brownies, and rice pudding whilst on a low carb routine, you simply need to tweak things to make them suitable for your new lifestyle change. Below you'll find a range of delicious desserts that you can make whenever you feel like adding something sweet to your day. Remember to watch the net carb amount and add this to the rest of your meals, but overall, many of the desserts below are relatively low in carbs anyway.

Low Carb Hot Chocolate

Serves 1
Fat – 23g, Net carbs – 1g, Protein – 1g, Calories – 216

INGREDIENTS

- ◆ 1 tbsp cocoa powder
- ◆ 240ml boiling water
- ◆ 28g butter
- ◆ 2.5 tsp powdered erythritol
- ◆ Quarter tsp vanilla extract

METHOD

1. Place all ingredients in a blender
2. Combine for around 20 seconds, until everything is mixed together well and you can see a foam appearing on the top
3. Pour into cups and serve immediately

Low Carb Brownies

Serves 24
Fat – 11g, Net carbs – 1g, Protein – 3g, Calories – 120

INGREDIENTS

- 80ml almond butter
- 170g softened butter
- 3 medium eggs
- 30g cocoa powder
- 160g erythritol
- 110g almond flour
- Half tsp coffee powder, instant variety
- 28g chopped dark chocolate
- Half tsp baking powder
- Half tsp salt
- 1 tbsp vanilla extract
- 2 tbsp water

METHOD

1. Take a large baking dish and line with parchment paper
2. Preheat the oven to 175°C
3. Use a hand mixer to combine the almond butter, eggs, butter, and erythritol, until everything is thoroughly mixed
4. Add the baking powder, cocoa powder, almond flour, vanilla, water, salt and coffee powder and combine once more until everything is well mixed

5. Add the chocolate and combine
6. Transfer the mixture to the baking dish and even out the top section
7. Bake for 25 minutes and allow to cool for half an hour before cutting into squares

Creamy Lemon Ice Cream

Serves 6
Fat – 27g, Net carbs – 3g, Protein – 5g, Calories – 270

INGREDIENTS

- 3 medium eggs
- 425g double cream
- The zest and juice of 1 lemon
- 70g erythritol

METHOD

1. Separate the eggs into two separate bowls
2. Beat the egg whites until they form a stiff consistency
3. Add the erythritol to the egg yolks and beat together until they create a light consistency
4. Add the juice from the lemon and combine once more
5. Fold the egg whites into the yolks slowly and carefully
6. Take a separate mixing bowl and add the cream, whipping until you see peaks forming
7. Carefully fold the eggs into the cream mixture, until everything is combined
8. Transfer the bowl to the freezer and freeze for around 2 hours
9. Make sure you check on the ice cream every half an hour and give it a stir

Decadent Chocolate Mousse

Serves 6
Fat – 27g, Net carbs – 4g, Protein – 3g, Calories – 256

INGREDIENTS

- 3 tbsp cocoa powder
- 750g coconut milk (canned)
- 1 tsp erythritol
- 1 tsp vanilla extract

METHOD

1. Refrigerate the coconut milk for around 4 hours, to allow the water to separate from the cream
2. Remove the cream from the can and place into a large mixing bowl. You can discard the water or use it for something else
3. Add the vanilla and erythritol to the bowl and combine everything well with a hand mixer. The mixture should be quite thick and smooth
4. Add the cocoa powder and keep mixing until everything is combined well and the mixture is thick
5. Divide into serving bowls

Low Carb Key Lime Pie

Serves 8
Fat – 36g, Net carbs – 8g, Protein – 6g, Calories – 371

INGREDIENTS

- 45g erythritol (powdered) – for the meringue
- 3 egg whites
- 55g chopped macadamia nuts
- Half tsp cream of tartar
- 1 tsp vanilla extract and 1 extra tsp for the filling
- A pinch of salt
- 65g erythritol (powdered) – for the filling
- 110g softened butter
- The zest of 6 limes
- 120ml lime juice
- 6 egg yolks
- 350ml double cream

METHOD

1. First, make the meringue crust. Take a 9 inch pie pan and grease with butter
2. Preheat your oven to 150°C
3. Take a medium mixing bowl and combine the cream of tartar, salt and egg whites with a hand mixer
4. Add 45g powdered erythritol and vanilla and continue to whisk until you see peaks forming

5. Use a spatula to fold in the nuts
6. Transfer the mixture to the pie pan and cover the entire pan, including the sides
7. Place in the oven and bake for 45 minutes
8. Allow the meringue to cool
9. Take a medium saucepan and add the butter, melting over a low heat
10. Add in the rest of the erythritol, lime zest and juice, combining well
11. Add the egg yolks and whisk
12. Allow the mixture to thicken, but keep whisking
13. Once thick, remove the pan from the heat and use a sieve to get rid of the lime zest
14. Place the mixture in the refrigerator for an hour
15. Take another mixing bowl and add the cream, using a hand mixer to thicken it
16. Add the vanilla and keep mixing until thickened
17. Fold the cream into the lime mixture and combine well
18. Transfer the cream mixture into the crust and smooth over to fill to all edges
19. Refrigerate overnight, or for at least 4 hours

No Need to Bake Chocolate Cake!

Serves 12

Fat – 39g, Net carbs – 4g, Protein – 8g, Calories – 405

INGREDIENTS

- 200g dark chocolate, sugar-free
- 300ml double cream
- 100g butter
- 100g pumpkin seeds
- 3 tbsp erythritol
- 200g chopped hazelnuts
- A pinch of salt

METHOD

1. Take a medium saucepan and add the cream and erythritol, combining well

2. Allow the mixture to simmer for a few minutes, until the mixture turns thicker

3. Remove from the heat and place to one side

4. Add the butter and chocolate into the mixture, adding the salt and combining well

5. Make sure everything is melted

6. Take a frying pan and add the pumpkin seeds and hazelnuts, cooking for a few minutes until golden

7. Chop the nuts once more and then ad most of them to the creamed mixture

8. Take an 8 inch springform pan and line with parchment paper
9. Transfer the mixture into the pan and smooth over
10. Sprinkle the rest of the nuts over the top
11. Cover the top of the cake with clingfilm and place in the refrigerator for one hour

Peanut Butter Cheesecake

Serves 16

Fat – 35g, Net carbs – 5g, Protein – 8g, Calories – 368

INGREDIENTS

- 1 medium egg (for the crust)
- 85g butter
- 55g erythritol
- 2 tbsp cocoa powder
- 170g almond flour
- 240ml sour cream
- 3 medium eggs (for the filling)
- 550g cream cheese
- 120ml peanut butter (smooth version)
- Half a tsp vanilla extract
- 1 tbsp coconut oil
- 60g dark chocolate, sugar-free

METHOD

1. Take a 9 inch springform pan and grease the inside
2. Preheat the oven to 150°C
3. Take a medium sized mixing bowl and add the butter, 1 egg, 60ml erythritol, cocoa powder, and almond flour, combining well
4. Transfer the mixture to the springform pan and press into the bottom
5. Place in the oven and bake for 10 minutes, before placing to one side

6. Take another mixing bowl and add the sour cream, the rest of the eggs, cream cheese, and combing well

7. Add the peanut butter, the rest of the erythritol, and the vanilla extract, combining everything well

8. Transfer the filling over the crust and spread from edge to edge

9. Place in the oven for 10 minutes. After 10 minutes, turn the oven down to 100°C and cook for another 25 minutes

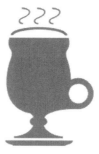

Berry Coconut Cream

Serves 1
Fat – 42g, Net carbs – 9g, Protein – 5g, Calories – 425

INGREDIENTS

- ♦ 55g strawberries, fresh
- ♦ 120ml coconut cream
- ♦ 1 tsp vanilla extract

METHOD

1. Place all ingredients in a large mixing bowl
2. Use a hand mixer or immersion blender to combine everything together until smooth
3. Serve in a tall glass, decorated with a spare strawberry or two!

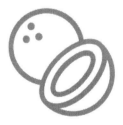

Luxurious Rice Pudding

Serves 6
Fat – 20g, Net carbs – 4g, Protein – 7g, Calories – 221

INGREDIENTS

- 300ml double cream
- 325ml cottage cheese
- 55g fresh berries (your choice)
- 1 tsp cinnamon, ground
- 1 tsp vanilla extract

METHOD

1. Take a large mixing bowl and add the cream, whipping with hand mixer until you see peaks forming
2. Add the vanilla and continue mixing
3. Use a spatula to fold in the cottage cheese carefully
4. Place the bowl in the refrigerator for around 15 minutes
5. Serve the pudding in bowls with berries on top and a sprinkle of cinnamon

Rich Berry Cobbler

Serves 4
Fat – 27g, Net carbs – 5g, Protein – 9g, Calories – 303

INGREDIENTS

- ◆ 55g almond flour
- ◆ 25g coconut flour
- ◆ 1 medium egg
- ◆ 280g blackberries, fresh work best
- ◆ 2 tbsp lime juice
- ◆ 2 tbsp powdered erythritol
- ◆ 85g butter

METHOD

1. Take a medium sized pie dish and preheat your oven to 175°C
2. Add the berries into the pie dish and distribute evenly
3. Squeeze the lime juice on top and give everything a stir
4. Take a medium bowl and add (apart from the butter) the rest of the ingredients, combining well until you get a crumbly consistency
5. Scatter the mixture over the top of the berries, covering as much as possible
6. Slice the butter into thin slices and add it on top of the cobbler
7. Place in the oven and cook for 15 minutes, until the top is browned

Now you've seen just how delicious following a low carb diet can be, it's time to start your journey. In this section, you'll find 14 days of meal plans, aimed towards making the start of your low carb route much easier to follow.

Of course, you can mix things up if you prefer to, especially if there is a dish that you don't like due to one of the ingredients. However, it's best to stick to the meal plans if you can, as that will ensure that you don't accidentally go over the recommended amount of carbs per day. By doing this, you'll lose weight faster and it will stay off. The plus point? You won't be hungry!

In the plans below you'll see that we've used recipes from the suggestions we've already given you, and each day has a new recipe to try too. This means you can expand your low carb repertoire even more!

You can add a dessert to your day if you want but remember to check that you're not going over your carb allowance. Aim for between 50 to 100 net carbs per day and you're within the range for weight loss. Remember to drink plenty of water and do exercise regularly too; that way, when you follow the meal plan below, you'll notice the numbers on the scales decreasing pretty quickly, and staying that way too.

Day 1

Breakfast: Easy bacon & eggs (See page 18)

Lunch: Mini Stuffed Peppers

Serves 4

Fat – 38g, Net carbs – 7g, Protein – 12g, Calories – 411

INGREDIENTS

- 28g chopped chorizo
- 230g mini bell peppers
- 230g cream cheese
- 110g grated cheddar cheese
- 1 tbsp thyme, fresh
- Half a tbsp chipotle paste
- 2 tbsp olive oil

METHOD

1. Cut your bell peppers lengthwise and remove the central core piece
2. Preheat your oven to 200°C
3. Take a small mixing bowl and add the cream cheese and all the pieces, combining well
4. Add the chopped chorizo and herbs to the bowl and combine well
5. Spoon the mixture into the peppers and fill to almost the top
6. Take a large baking dish and grease it with a little oil

7. Add the peppers to the baking dish, leaving a little space in-between
8. Sprinkle the cheddar over the top of the peppers
9. Bake for 20 minutes, checking after 15 minutes to ensure they're not burning

Dinner: Fragrant garlic chicken (See page 44)

Day 2

Breakfast: Cauliflower breakfast pancakes (See page 27)

Lunch: Traditional Caesar salad (See page 30)

Dinner: Meatballs With Onion Gravy

Serves 4

Fat – 71g, Net carbs – 16g, Protein – 42g, Calories – 880

INGREDIENTS

- 650g ground beef
- 60ml double cream for the patties
- 1 medium egg
- 1 minced onion
- 3 tbsp butter for frying the meat
- 1 tsp salt
- Half a tsp black pepper
- 3 sliced onions (very thinly sliced)
- 2 tbsp butter for the gravy
- 325ml double cream from the gravy
- Half a tbsp of soy sauce
- 450g broccoli

METHOD

1. Take a large mixing bowl and add the beef, breaking it up as much as you can
2. Add the cream, onion, egg, and the spices and combine everything well

3. Delve into the bowl with your hands and create patties, flattening them down

4. Take a large frying pan and melt the butter

5. Cook the patties on each side for around 3 minutes

6. Take a large ovenproof dish and transfer the patties into the dish, retaining the juices from the frying pan

7. Cook in the oven at 100°C as you complete the recipe

8. Transfer the juices from the frying pan into a mixing jug and add just enough water to loosen it

9. Take a medium frying pan and add a little butter to fry the onions until they're soft

10. Take a medium saucepan and add the meat juices and the cream, combining together

11. Add the rest of the ingredients, apart from the broccoli, and combine

12. Bring the contents of the pan to the boil and then turn down to a simmer for around 10 minutes, until thickened slightly

13. Add the onions and combine, seasoning with a little salt and pepper

14. Cut the broccoli into small florets and boil in some salted water until they're to your liking

15. Drain the broccoli and let it cool a little

16. Remove the patties from the oven and arrange on your plate, pouring the onion gravy over the top and serving the broccoli on the side

Day 3

Breakfast: Homemade Granola
Serves 20
Fat – 29g, Net carbs – 7g, Protein – 16g, Calories – 356

INGREDIENTS

- 55g almond flour
- 4 tbsp coconut oil
- 240ml water
- 230g pecan nuts
- 140g sunflower seeds
- 70g finely shredded coconut
- 1 tbsp turmeric
- 1 tbsp cinnamon, ground
- 2 tsp vanilla extract
- 130g flaxseed
- 4 tbsp pumpkin seeds
- 4 tbsp sesame seeds

METHOD

1. Place all the nuts into a food processer and blitz until they're coarsely chopped
2. Preheat your oven to 150°C
3. Place all the ingredients into a large mixing bowl and combine really well
4. Take a baking sheet and line it with parchment paper

5. Transfer the mixture onto the parchment paper and arrange it into one even layer

6. Place in the oven for 20 minutes, but check halfway to ensure the nuts aren't starting to burn

7. Remove the sheet from the oven and give everything a really good stir

8. Return to the oven for another 20 minutes

9. The granola is cooked when everything has a dry feel to it

10. Remove the sheet from the oven and allow to cool completely

11. Serve your granola with cream or Greek yogurt, according to your liking

Lunch: Tuna & boiled eggs (See page 33)

Dinner: Low carb chicken korma (See page 45)

Day 4

Breakfast: Buttery scrambled eggs (See page 19)

Lunch: Healthy avocado & salmon (See page 32)

Dinner: Blue Cheese Chicken Wings

Serves 4

Fat – 67g, Net carbs – 4g, Protein – 50g, Calories – 830

INGREDIENTS

- ♦ 900g chicken wings
- ♦ 80ml mayonnaise
- ♦ 3 tsp lemon juice
- ♦ 60ml sour cream
- ♦ 60ml double cream
- ♦ 85g crumbled blue cheese
- ♦ Half a tsp garlic powder, plus another half a tsp for the chicken
- ♦ Half a tsp salt
- ♦ 2 tbsp olive oil
- ♦ 1 garlic clove, minced
- ♦ Quarter tsp black pepper
- ♦ 40g grated parmesan cheese
- ♦ 30g stalks of celery

1. Take a large mixing bowl and add the sour cream, mayonnaise, lemon juice quarter of a teaspoon of garlic powder, double cream and a pinch of salt. Combine everything well

2. Crumble the blue cheese into the bowl and combine once more

3. Place the dip in the refrigerator for around 45 minutes to 1 hour

4. Take a large bowl and add the chicken wings

5. Add the spices and the oil and combine everything really well

6. Place the chicken into the refrigerator for half an hour

7. Preheat your oven to 200°C

8. Place the chicken onto a large baking sheet and bake for half an hour, checking the chicken is thoroughly cooked through

9. Take another large bowl and add the parmesan and the chicken, combing everything until really well coated

10. Place the chicken onto a plate. Serve with the blue cheese zip on the side, and celery sticks for dipping

Day 5

Breakfast: Egg muffins (See page 28)

Lunch: Shrimp Ceviche
Serves 4
Fat – 9g, Net carbs – 6g, Protein – 17g, Calories – 181

INGREDIENTS

- 450g shelled and deveined shrimp
- 1 cucumber
- Half a red onion, cut into large strips
- 240ml lemon juice
- 14g coriander
- 1 avocado, pitted and sliced
- 1 deseeded jalapeno
- Salt and pepper for seasoning

METHOD

1. Take a large bowl and add the shrimp
2. Add most of the lemon juice into the bowl and combine
3. Place the bowl into the refrigerator for half an hour
4. Take the cucumber and remove the skin, cutting it into two, lengthwise and then creating smaller strips
5. Take your blender and add the jalapeno, coriander, and the remaining lemon juice, combining well with a little salt and pepper. Place the sauce to one side when it has created a smooth sauce
6. Place the sauce into a medium sized serving bowl

7. Take the shrimp out of the bowl and shake to remove the excess lemon
8. Drizzle a very small amount of the lemon juice over the top
9. Add the onion and the cucumber to the bowl and mix slightly
10. Decorate with avocado and enjoy

Dinner: Lasagne with courgette (See page 47)

Day 6

Breakfast: Chia Almond Butter Pancakes
Serves 2
Fat – 48g, Net carbs – 5g, Protein – 17g, Calories – 562

INGREDIENTS

- 2 tsp psyllium husk powder, ground
- 50g crushed chia seeds
- 180ml almond milk
- 1 tsp vanilla extract
- 3 tbsp protein powder, unflavoured
- Half a tsp baking powder
- A pinch of salt
- Quarter of a tsp ground cinnamon
- 3 tbsp melted almond butter
- 4 tbsp coconut oil

METHOD

1. Take a large bowl and combine the chia seeds, protein powder, psyllium husk powder, baking powder, salt, and cinnamon

2. Add the almond butter, vanilla and almond milk and combine until you get a quite chick consistency batter

3. Take a large frying pan and add the coconut oil over a medium heat

4. When the pan is hot, add around 4 tablespoons of the mixture into the pan, to create a round shape
5. Cook for around 4 minutes on each side and flip over halfway
6. Cook for another 2 minutes on the other side

Lunch: Halloumi with mushrooms (See page 34)

Dinner: Goat's cheese & spinach dinner pie (See page 49)

Day 7

Breakfast: Fruity strawberry breakfast smoothie (See page 21)

Lunch: Avocado & tuna salad (See page 35)

Dinner: Traditional Shepherd's Pie

Serves 4

Fat – 36g, Net carbs – 15g, Protein – 37g, Calories – 555

INGREDIENTS

- 650g ground beef
- 3 onions
- 3 cloves of garlic
- 3 carrots
- 450g cauliflower
- 60ml olive oil
- 260g cherry tomatoes
- Salt and pepper for seasoning

METHOD

1. Take a large baking dish and preheat your oven to 175°C
2. Create florets out of the cauliflower and cuts the tomatoes into halves. Also, create small cubes out of the carrots and onions
3. Take a large saucepan and add a little salt. Add the garlic, oil, cauliflower and season once more
4. Cook the cauliflower until it is tender and remove from the heat
5. Take a large frying pan and add a little oil over a medium heat
6. Add the onions and carrot san cook until soft

7. Add the beef and combine, breaking it up well

8. Season and cook until the meat is brown

9. Add the tomatoes to the pan and cook for another 3 minutes

10. Transfer the mixture to the baking dish and spread out into an even layer

11. Drain the cauliflower and place the pot you cooked the cauliflower in, back on the stove over a medium heat

12. Return the cauliflower to the pot and add a little oil, cooking for a few minutes

13. Use a potato masher to create cauliflower mash, as smooth as you can get it

14. Add the mash over the top of the meat mixture and create an even layer

15. Place the dish into the oven for 20 minutes, until brown and crisp on top

Day 8

Breakfast: Classic huevos rancheros (See page 20)

Lunch: Low Carb Burgers
Serves 4
Fat – 85g, Net carbs – 6g, Protein – 54g, Calories – 1049

INGREDIENTS

- 140g almond flour
- 2 tsp baking powder
- 5 tbsp psyllium husk powder
- 300ml water
- 2 tsp cider vinegar
- 3 egg whites
- 1 tbsp sesame seeds
- 2 tbsp butter
- 800g ground beef
- 55g shredded lettuce
- 1 thinly sliced tomato
- 1 thinly sliced onion
- 140g bacon
- 120ml mayonnaise
- Salt and pepper for seasoning

1. First, you're going to make low carb burger buns. Preheat your oven to 175°C

2. Take a large mixing bowl and add the almond flour, psyllium husk powder, baking powder sesame seeds, and a little salt. Combine everything well

3. Boil the water and add it to the bowl, along with the egg whites and vinegar, beating for half a minute with a hand mixture

4. Create four equally sized buns out of the dough, using your hands

5. Take a baking sheet and line with parchment paper

6. Add the dough to the parchment and leave a little room between each one

7. Place in the oven for around 50 minutes, checking if they're done before removing. If not, bake for another 10 minutes

8. Meanwhile, cook the bacon to your liking

9. Place the ground beef into a bowl and use your hands to form four hamburgers

10. Take a large frying pan and use a little oil to fry the burgers, seasoning with salt and pepper as you go

11. Flip the burgers after around 10 minutes and cook on the other side

12. Cut each of the burger buns in half and spread mayonnaise on each

13. Place the lettuce on one side of the buns

14. Place the burger onto the bun

15. Add the tomato and the onion

16. Top with the other half of the bun

Dinner: Creamy cauliflower cheese (See page 51)

Day 9

Breakfast: Cheesy scrambled eggs with spinach (See page 22)

Lunch: Healthy green beans with salmon (See page 37)

Dinner: Bacon & Ranch Chicken

Serves 6

Fat – 35g, Net carbs – 3g, Protein – 45g, Calories – 519

INGREDIENTS

- 900g chicken breasts
- 1 tbsp ranch seasoning
- 280g cream cheese
- 140g diced bacon
- 2 tbsp chopped chives
- 90g baby spinach
- 110g cheddar cheese
- Salt and pepper for seasoning

METHOD

1. Take a medium mixing bowl and combine the cream cheese and ranch seasoning. Add a little salt and combine once more
2. Take a slow cooker and arrange the chicken at the bottom of the cooker
3. Spread the cheese mixture over the top of the chicken
4. Place the lid on the slow cooker and cook for 3 hours on a high setting

5. Cook the bacon to your liking and place to one side
6. Once the chicken is cooked, use two forks to shred into pieces
7. Take a large mixing bowl and place everything inside, combining well
8. Add the cheese and place under the grill to allow the cheese to melt
9. Season and serve with the chives over the top and baby spinach to the side

Day 10

Breakfast: Healthy Ginger Smoothie
Serves 2
Fat – 8g, Net carbs – 3g, Protein – 1g, Calories – 83

INGREDIENTS

- 160ml water
- 28g spinach, frozen works well
- 80ml coconut milk
- 2 tbsp lime juice
- 2 tsp grated ginger
- Extra grated ginger for decoration

METHOD

1. Take a blender and add the water, grated ginger, spinach, and coconut milk inside
2. Add half of the lime juice and combine everything until it forms a smooth consistency
3. Pour the smoothie into glasses
4. Add a little grated ginger over the top for decoration and enjoy

Lunch: Tasty baked eggs (See page 36)
Dinner: Low carb chowder (See page 53)

Day 11

Breakfast: Spinach breakfast frittata (See page 23)

Lunch: Leek & Broccoli Soup With Cheese Crisps
Serves 4
Fat – 53g, Net carbs – 11g, Protein – 17g, Calories – 588

INGREDIENTS

- 300g broccoli
- 1 leek
- 1 vegetable stock cube
- 475ml water
- 21g chopped basil
- 1 pressed garlic clove
- 200g cream cheese
- 240ml double cream
- 170g grated cheddar cheese
- Half a tsp paprika
- Salt and pepper for seasoning

METHOD

1. Take the leek and chop into small pieces
2. Cut the broccoli into florets and retain half, with the other half to one side
3. Chop one half of the florets very thinly
4. Take a large saucepan and add the chopped broccoli and leeks
5. Add the water until it covers the mixture

6. Add the vegetable stock cube and season

7. Bring the pot to the boil and then turn down to simmer until the broccoli is soft

8. Add the rest of the broccoli to the pot and combine

9. Lower the heat to a simmer

10. Add the cream, cream cheese, garlic and basil, seasoning a little and combine

11. Use a hand blender to create a smooth consistency

12. Create the cheese crisps by taking a baking sheet and lining it with parchment paper

13. Create mounds of grated cheese on the parchment paper, leaving a little space between

14. Sprinkle a little paprika on top and place in the oven for around 5 minutes

15. Once they've cooled slightly, the crisps will be harder

Dinner: Creamy tuna casserole (See page 55)

Day 12

Breakfast: Breakfast Chia Pudding
Serves 1
Fat – 56g, Net carbs – 8g, Protein – 9g, Calories – 568

INGREDIENTS

- 2 tbsp chia seeds
- Half a tsp vanilla extract
- 240ml coconut milk

METHOD

1. Take a glass mixing jug and add all ingredients
2. Combine well
3. Cover the top of the jug with a lid or plastic wrap and place in the refrigerator overnight
4. Serve the next morning

Lunch: Lunchtime chicken soup (See page 38)

Dinner: Meatball & bacon casserole (See page 57)

Day 13

Breakfast: Blueberry pancakes (See page 24)

Lunch: Halloumi bacon wraps (See page 40)

Dinner: Thai-Style Curry

Serves 4

Fat – 74g, Net carbs – 10g, Protein – 42g, Calories – 867

INGREDIENTS

- 650g boneless salmon fillets
- 1 tbsp coconut oil
- 28g butter
- 475ml coconut cream
- 450g cauliflower
- 2 tbsp red curry paste
- 8g chopped coriander
- Salt and pepper for seasoning

METHOD

1. Take a medium baking dish and grease with a little butter
2. Preheat your oven to 200°C
3. Arrange the fish in the baking dish and season
4. Place a little button on top of each fillet
5. Take a small mixing bowl and combine the curry paste, coriander and coconut cream

6. Pour the mixture over the fish
7. Place in the oven for around 20 minutes
8. Cut the cauliflower into florets
9. Take a medium saucepan and boil the cauliflower in salted water for 2-3 minutes
10. Serve the cauliflower beside the curry

Day 14

Breakfast: Cheesy omelette (See page 26)

Lunch: Beef Salad, Asian-Style
Serves 2
Fat – 72g, Net carbs – 8g, Protein – 48g, Calories – 873

INGREDIENTS

- 1 tsp sesame oil for the mayonnaise
- 80ml mayonnaise
- Half a tbsp lime juice
- 1 tbsp olive oil
- 1 tbsp grated ginger
- 1 tbsp fish sauce
- 450g steak, ribeye works well
- 1 tsp chilli flakes
- 6 halved cherry tomatoes
- 85g chopped lettuce
- 55g chopped cucumber
- Half a chopped red onion
- 1 tsp sesame seeds
- 2 chopped scallions
- 8g chopped coriander

1. Take a medium mixing bowl and add the mayonnaise, lime juice and season with a little salt and pepper, combining well. Place this to one side

2. Take a large mixing bowl and add the olive oil, fish sauce, grated ginger, steak, and chilli flakes, combining well

3. Pour this mixture into a plastic bag. Place in the refrigerator for 15minutes

4. Arrange the coriander, onion, lettuce, cucumber, and tomatoes onto two plates

5. Take a medium frying pan and add the sesame seeds, toasting for around 2 minutes

6. Take the meat and pat dry

7. Remove the sesame seeds from the pan and set to one side

8. Add the meat to the pan and cook on each side for two minutes

9. Turn the heat down and cook until it is to your liking

10. Remove the meat and place on a cutting board, slicing into pieces

11. Add the scallions to the pan and cook for a couple of minutes

12. Add the beef on top of the vegetables on the plate, and then the scallions

13. Add the sesame seeds and the mayonnaise before serving

Dinner: Homemade low carb pizza (See page 59)

CONCLUSION

And that's how you do low carb!

If you thought it would be a hard lifestyle change to follow, you're hopefully now quite clear about how easy low carb really is. It's packed with delicious meals and snacks that you can enjoy every single day.

The high fat amount in your day will also mean that you're full and not craving everything under the sun.

That's the reason why so many fad diets don't work. You're just not full and as a result, you're craving things. When you crave for long enough, you're sure to give in. This often leads to binge eating and then you shrug your shoulders and wonder why you should carry on. The guilt cycle that follows trying and failing at a fad diet is extreme. For this reason, steer clear of fad diets and focus on healthy lifestyle changes instead.

When you lower a crucial nutritional group, it's normal to worry that it's not safe. However, as long as you get enough fat in your diet and you have enough protein too, low carb is perfectly safe. However, if you have any health concerns or you have diabetes and you're taking medication, be sur to check things out with your doctor first. Also remember, if you're pregnant or breastfeeding, low carb may not be the route for you right now – talk to your doctor for expert advice on this.

You'll quickly see that following a low carb diet is far more sustainable than any other diet you've tried in the past. You'll also notice that any weight you lose will stay off, rather than coming back as soon as you start to eat slightly more "normally".

Drink plenty of water and do more exercise alongside your new lifestyle change and your health will improve for the better.

All you need to do now is decide which delicious recipe you're going to try first!

Move into your new low carb lifestyle with positivity and expect results. There is no reason why weight loss won't come your way if you keep that fat burning switch firmly on. With no cravings and delicious homemade meals to look forward to every day, you'll be smiling and healthy at the same time. What's better than that?

DISCLAIMER

This book contains opinions and ideas of the author and is meant to teach the reader informative and helpful knowledge while due care should be taken by the user in the application of the information provided. The instructions and strategies are possibly not right for every reader and there is no guarantee that they work for everyone. Using this book and implementing the information/recipes therein contained is explicitly your own responsibility and risk. This work with all its contents, does not guarantee correctness, completion, quality or correctness of the provided information. Misinformation or misprints cannot be completely eliminated.

Printed in Great Britain
by Amazon